Introduction

This book covers some of the most common health and safety issues in the workplace. Many improvements can be made by taking simple steps to reduce the effects equipment, the working environment and specific tasks have on health and safety.

Everyone plays an important part in safety at work. This book will help you to carry out your work activities more safely and in a way that protects your health. The book will also help you to understand the principles behind those health and safety issues with which you are not directly involved.

In some circumstances, even the decision-makers for your workplace need additional advice and information. In cases of a technical nature or where severe hazards exist, expert advice from suitably-qualified and experienced professionals is required.

An Introduction to Health and Safety in Health and Social Care focuses on good practice. It is not intended as a complete or authoritative guide to the law – employers, managers and the self-employed will require further information. Advice and information can be obtained from the relevant enforcement authority.

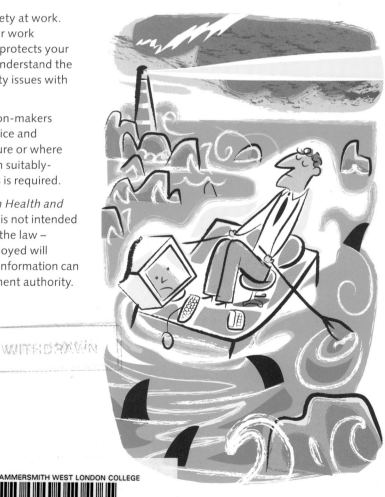

Chapter 1
A background to health and safety in health and social care

Health and safety at work describes measures designed to protect the health and safety of people at work and that of others, such as patients, clients, visitors and members of the public, who are affected by work activities.

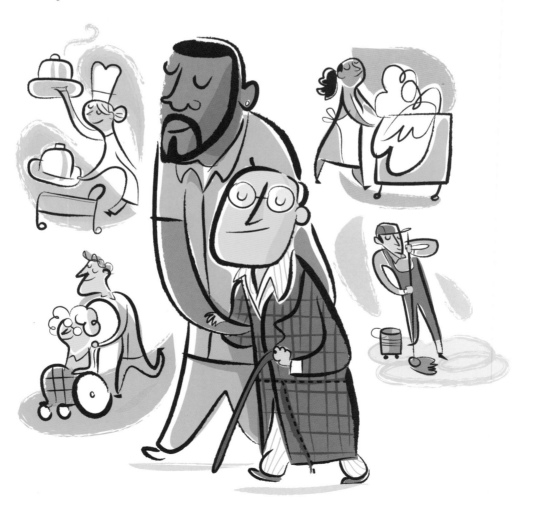

Key words

Accident – an unplanned, uncontrolled event with the potential to cause injury, damage or other loss.

Hazard – something with the potential to cause harm.

Health – a state of well-being, with the absence of illness or disease.

Health and Safety Executive (HSE) – the body that regulates health and safety and a major enforcement authority.

Health and safety policy – a document outlining an employer's general policy and commitment to health and safety. It will also include an outline of the organisation and people's responsibilities, together with arrangements for implementing the policy.

Occupational illness – health problems associated with work.

Risk – the chance (or likelihood) that a hazard will cause harm. In assessing the risk, consideration needs to be given to the degree of harm and the number of people who may be affected.

Safety – the absence of risks.

Workplace – any building or area where people work.

Workplace accidents and illness

There are hundreds of thousands of accidents in the workplace every year. In Britain alone, it has been estimated that 2.3 million people suffer work-related ill health.

Official figures for workplace injuries in Britain in the year 2003 to 2004 show that there were:

- 606 fatalities

- 45,516 major injuries

- 130,247 injuries leading to more than three days' absence from work.

The statistics for fatal and major injuries cover members of the public as well as employees and self-employed people. The figures for absences of longer than three days relate to employees. In reality, the figures are likely to be much higher because many accidents are not reported formally.

Fatal accidents are most commonly caused by:
- falls from height (67)

- being struck by a moving object or vehicle (44)

- being struck by a moving, flying or falling object (29).

Major injury accidents are most commonly caused by:
- slipping, tripping or falling (11,269)

- falls from height (3,884)

- handling, lifting or carrying (4,324).

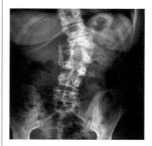

Slips, trips and falls are a common cause of major injury

Absences of over three days are most commonly caused by:

- being injured while handling, lifting or carrying (52,422)

- slips, trips and falls (30,049)

- being struck by a moving, flying or falling object (14,780).

Other categories of accidents include:

- coming into contact with moving machinery

- coming into contact with harmful substances, such as chemicals

- making contact with electricity

- being injured by a patient or client (work-related violence)

- becoming trapped

- various effects of fire, such as heat and smoke

- explosion.

Occupational illnesses – those linked to work activities or the workplace – include diseases and conditions, such as:

- stress, depression and anxiety

- musculoskeletal disorders

- breathing and lung illnesses, e.g. asthma

- skin diseases, e.g. dermatitis

- infections

- hearing damage

- vibration injuries.

Reducing accidents and ill health in the health and social care sectors will:

- protect the health and livelihoods of workers

- improve the quality of care provision

- save NHS, social services and private sector money.

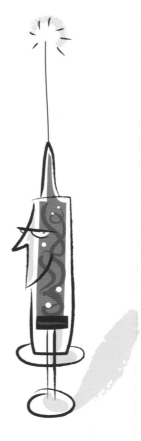

Key points

- Accidents are frequently caused by:

  - poor lifting and carrying

  - slips, trips and falls

  - being hit by moving objects or vehicles

  - misuse of moving machinery

  - using harmful substances incorrectly

  - using sharp objects

  - not following instructions.

- Health and social care workers can be exposed to a variety of health and safety hazards.

The costs of accidents and illness

Accidents and illness cause a great deal of personal pain and suffering for individuals, as well as worry and financial difficulty for families. Employers have to provide temporary cover during staff absence and can lose money as a result of disrupted care and treatment. In health and social care, this equates to a reduction in efficiency and a detrimental effect on funding and cash management. A study by the Health and Safety Executive (HSE) showed that accidents can cost up to 37% of an organisation's profits.

Accidents and ill health can also be expensive for society as a whole. Another HSE study estimated an annual cost to society of between £20 billion and £31.8 billion, including medical costs, lost days' work and sick pay.

While there are certainly some direct costs involved in developing good health and safety standards at work – for example, in providing training and new equipment, there are huge potential long-term savings that can benefit individuals, families, companies and society as a whole.

Costs of poor health and safety standards

- Accidents, illness and stress.
- Deaths.
- Increased sick leave.
- Loss of production.
- Loss of earnings and increased personal costs.
- Bad publicity, resulting in a loss of reputation.
- Lowered staff performance and morale.
- Reduced organisational performance.
- High staff turnover.
- Prosecution, fines and imprisonment.
- Prohibition and closure.
- Compensation claims.
- Increased insurance costs.
- Legal costs.
- Loss of jobs.
- Treatment costs – first aid, etc.
- Costs to the health service and society as a whole.

Benefits of good health and safety standards

- Healthy, happy and motivated work teams.
- A safer working environment.
- Fewer accidents.
- Reduction in sick leave.
- Professional reputation.
- Increased performance and standards conformance.
- Orderly working environment and procedures.
- Confidence in health and safety standards.
- Increased job security.
- Lower insurance premiums.
- Less chance of civil actions and compensation claims.
- Less chance of prosecutions.

Key point

- Apart from causing pain and discomfort to people, accidents and illness also result in financial burdens on employers and society.

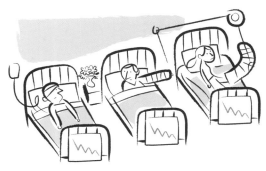

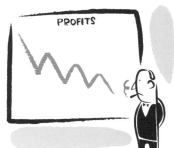

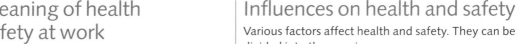

The meaning of health and safety at work

Most people spend a significant part of their lives at work and do not expect their health to be damaged through work-related illness, disease or injury. Health and safety measures are concerned with controlling and reducing risks to the health and safety of anyone who might be affected by work activities.

Influences on health and safety

Various factors affect health and safety. They can be divided into three main groups:

1. Occupational factors – people may be at risk from certain illnesses or injuries because of the work they do – for example, back strain from lifting people or heavy objects, or needlestick injuries from incorrect disposal of sharps.

2. Environmental factors – the conditions in which people work may cause problems, e.g. slippery or wet surfaces caused by water or other fluids.

3. Human factors – poor behaviour and attitudes can contribute to accidents, including error, carelessness, poor concentration, haste and ignorance of correct procedures.

Accidents may result from a combination of human error and faults in equipment or the working environment.

Key point

■ Health and safety is affected by occupational, environmental and human factors.

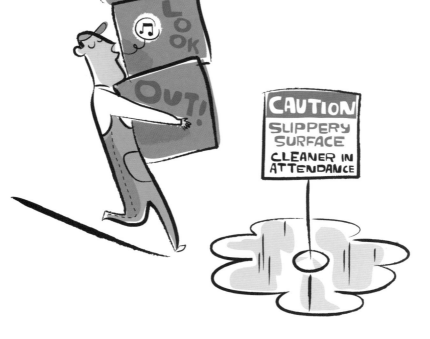

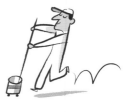

Achieving high standards

There will always be risks in the workplace, but they can be controlled by high standards of health and safety, such as:

- an effective management system and health and safety policy that set the standards and keep work activities under control

- good communication amongst everyone in the workplace and with other people that the organisation/business deals with

- positive attitudes towards health and safety, with everyone being involved and taking it seriously

- an effective risk assessment strategy aimed at reducing the likelihood of accidents and ill health

- buildings and equipment designed with health and safety in mind

- carrying out safe working practices

- good standards of cleaning and maintenance

- well informed and trained managers and staff

- an efficient reporting system for accidents, ill health and safety defects

- careful monitoring and the undertaking of remedial action to improve any deficiencies – a commitment to continual improvement in the workplace.

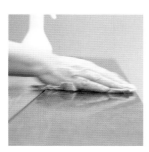 Good standards of cleaning and maintenance can help to reduce the risks to health and safety

Summary

1. Accidents are frequently caused by:

- poor lifting and carrying

- slips, trips and falls

- being hit by moving objects or vehicles

- misuse of moving machinery

- using harmful substances incorrectly

- using sharp objects

- not following instructions.

2. Health and social care workers can be exposed to a variety of health and safety hazards.

3. Apart from causing pain and discomfort to people, accidents and illness also result in financial burdens on employers and society.

4. Health and safety is affected by occupational, environmental and human factors.

5. Risks in the workplace can be controlled by effective standards of health and safety.

Key point

- Risks in the workplace can be controlled by effective standards of health and safety.

Chapter 2
Health and safety law

Most countries have developed legislation to protect the health and safety of people at work. In Britain, employers must take reasonable care to protect employees from the risks of injury, disease or death, while employees must take care to protect themselves and others who may be affected by their activities whilst at work.

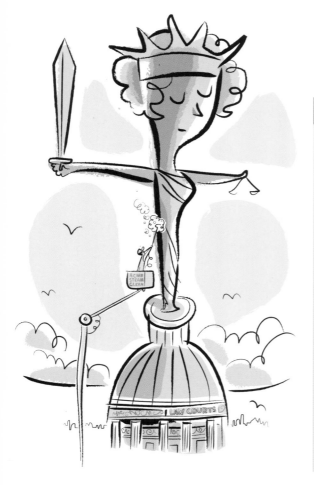

Key words

Directive – instructions from the European Union for member states to pass laws specifying certain standards.

Enforcement authority – the organisation responsible for enforcing health and safety legislation.

Enforcement officers – environmental health practitioners, health and safety inspectors and others who are responsible for enforcing legislation.

Environmental Health Practitioners (EHPs) – enforcement officers from local authorities.

Legislation – a general term for laws, including acts, regulations, orders and directives.

Local authority – the local council.

Reasonably practicable – a legal expression that balances risk against the time, trouble and money to prevent or reduce risk.

Welfare – issues concerning the well-being of employees, such as the provision of toilets.

Complying with the law

This chapter highlights some of the main issues that are controlled by health and safety legislation, although it does not cover every aspect of the law.

In 1991, the NHS lost its Crown Immunity and so now comes under the control of the enforcement authorities responsible for enforcing health and safety legislation in other sectors. Individual trust directors must comply with health and safety laws and take responsibility for employees, patients and clients, visitors and contractors – in fact, anyone who might be affected by the daily activities of their establishments.

It is the responsibility of employers, the self-employed and those with specific responsibilities for health and safety to ensure that they are familiar with all the relevant legal obligations affecting their workplace. They must also ensure that they are sufficiently informed, trained and qualified to make decisions aimed at achieving appropriate health and safety standards. This may involve obtaining specialist advice and help.

Some aspects of health and safety might be covered by more than one branch of a country's legal system. In Britain, for instance, this means that a *criminal* court can impose penalties, including fines and imprisonment, when an individual or a company breaks a law. In some cases, it is also possible for claims to be made through *civil* courts for financial compensation for harm, injury or damage.

Key point

- It is the responsibility of employers, the self-employed and those with specific responsibilities for health and safety to ensure that they are familiar with all the relevant legal obligations affecting their workplace.

Work-related legislation

Legislation covers a wide range of health and safety issues. Laws in Britain tend to focus on one of the following:

- particular types of workplace, such as factories and construction sites
- a specific topic affecting a variety of workplaces and work activities – *see* list below
- general issues that affect every workplace, such as the management of health and safety.

Among the subjects covered by specific legislation are:

- workplaces
- work equipment
- safety signs
- electricity
- fire
- working at height
- highly flammable liquids
- display screen equipment
- manual handling
- hazardous substances
- noise
- personal protective equipment
- first aid
- reporting of injuries, diseases and dangerous occurrences
- consultation with employees
- health and safety management.

Legal responsibilities

Employers, employees and other groups have specific legal responsibilities for health and safety at work. These duties are covered by The Health and Safety at Work etc. Act 1974 (in England, Wales and Scotland) and by The Health and Safety at Work (Northern Ireland) Order 1978. These give legal responsibilities to:

- employers
- employees
- the self-employed
- designers, manufacturers and suppliers
- people in control of work premises.

Employers' duties

Employers must ensure that the health, safety and welfare of employees are protected, so far as is reasonably practicable. In particular, employers must:

- provide and maintain equipment and work systems that are safe and healthy
- deal with substances, such as chemicals, sharps and other waste, safely
- provide information, instruction, training and supervision
- maintain safe and healthy workplaces with the necessary facilities
- provide a health and safety policy statement when employing five or more people.

They must also ensure that workplaces and work activities do not put visitors, members of the public and others at unnecessary risk.

Employees' duties

Employees also have legal responsibilities. They must:

- take care of their own health and safety at work
- take care of the health and safety of others
- co-operate with their employer
- report dangerous situations to their supervisor or employer
- not misuse or interfere with anything provided for health and safety purposes.

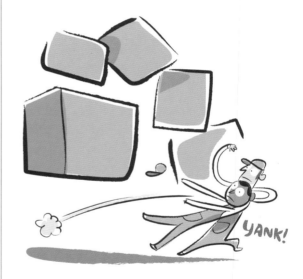

Duties of people in control of work premises

People who are in charge of a workplace have legal responsibilities to ensure safe and healthy premises.

Duties of the self-employed

Self-employed people have the legal duty not to put other people at risk by the way in which they work. This category of workers includes health and social care professionals who work on a freelance or contracted basis.

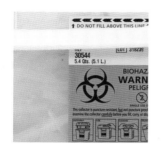

Always follow instructions for the safe use of equipment

Duties of designers, manufacturers, suppliers and installers

These groups have legal responsibilities for the design and construction of articles, the use of substances, and the testing and installation of their work. They must provide adequate information, such as instructions for the safe use of a machine. It is also the duty of management within the health and social care sectors to ensure that only competent (approved) suppliers are used.

Key points

- Everyone has legal responsibilities for health and safety at work.

- Employers, employees, the self-employed, designers, manufacturers, suppliers, installers and people in control of work premises have specific legal responsibilities.

- Employees must:

  - take care of their own health and safety at work

  - take care of the health and safety of others

  - co-operate with their employer

  - report dangerous situations to their supervisor or employer

  - not misuse or interfere with anything provided for health and safety purposes.

The management of health and safety at work

The Management of Health and Safety at Work Regulations 1999 (originally 1992) (in England, Wales and Scotland) and The Management of Health and Safety at Work Regulations (Northern Ireland) 2000 have had a major impact on the way companies and organisations control health and safety standards.

Employers must undertake a range of tasks, including:

- carrying out risk assessments (*see* Chapter 3)

- making arrangements for the planning, organisation, control, monitoring and review of health and safety measures

- appointing a competent person or persons to assist with health and safety

- establishing emergency procedures

- providing health and safety information and training.

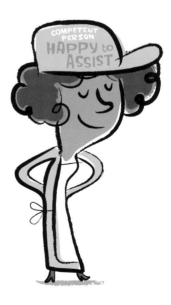

Enforcement

Enforcement officers help to ensure compliance with the law. The Health and Safety Executive (HSE) is the enforcement authority for premises, such as factories, in England, Scotland and Wales. In most of the service sector, which includes shops, offices and wholesale and catering premises, enforcement is carried out by environmental health practitioners (EHPs) or technical officers from the local authority.

Until the formation of the Health and Safety Executive for Northern Ireland in 1999, enforcement in the province was undertaken by the Health and Safety Inspectorate and the Health and Safety Agency.

In general terms hospitals are within the control of the HSE. Care homes that have a high level of nursing requirement also fall under their control. Homes that are mainly residential are generally inspected by the local authority – the only exception being where a residential home is operated by a local authority, then the HSE has responsibility for matters involving health and safety.

Enforcement officers have wide-ranging powers to help them to carry out their job. They can:

- enter premises
- conduct investigations
- take samples and photographs
- ask questions
- give advice
- issue instructions – improvement notices and prohibition notices (see below) – that must be carried out by law
- initiate a prosecution.

Employers are often given the opportunity of putting problems right before formal action is taken. This may be done by giving verbal or written advice, but it is sometimes necessary to serve a legal notice.

Improvement notices

These specify that certain actions must be taken within a specific period of time. For example, a damaged floor must be repaired to remove a tripping hazard.

Prohibition notices

These are issued where there is a risk of serious personal injury. The notice may require a particular activity to stop immediately, such as the use of a dangerous machine, or it could even result in the premises being closed down – that is, the suspension of care and treatment of patients or clients

Prosecution

Enforcement officers can start legal proceedings when offences have been committed. Prosecution is more likely when there is a serious health and safety problem or when somebody has ignored the officers' attempts to have health and safety deficiencies remedied. Prosecution is also likely if someone fails to comply with a notice.

Individuals, including company directors and members of staff, can be prosecuted as well as a corporate body, i.e. a company or organisation as a whole. Prosecution can result in unlimited fines, imprisonment for up to two years, or both.

Key points

- The powers of enforcement officers include entering premises, carrying out investigations and serving notices.
- Prosecution for breaching health and safety laws can result in unlimited fines, imprisonment for up to two years, or both.

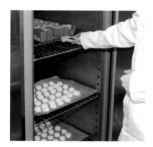

Enforcement officers can enter premises and conduct investigations

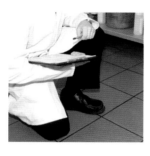

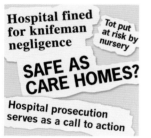

Breaching health and safety laws can result in fines and imprisonment

Summary

1. It is the responsibility of employers, the self-employed and those with specific responsibilities for health and safety to ensure that they are familiar with all the relevant legal obligations affecting their workplace.

2. Everyone has legal responsibilities for health and safety at work.

3. Employers, employees, the self-employed, designers, manufacturers, suppliers, installers and people in control of work premises have specific legal responsibilities.

4. Employees must:

- take care of their own health and safety at work

- take care of the health and safety of others

- co-operate with their employer

- report dangerous situations to their supervisor or employer

- not misuse or interfere with anything provided for health and safety purposes.

5. The powers of enforcement officers include entering premises, carrying out investigations and serving notices.

6. Prosecution for breaching health and safety laws can result in unlimited fines, imprisonment for up to two years, or both.

Chapter 3
Risk assessment

Risk assessment is a technique for preventing accidents and ill health by helping people to think about what could go wrong and ways to prevent problems. Risk assessment is good practice and a legal requirement. It often enables organisations to reduce the costs associated with accidents and ill health and to help them to decide their priorities, highlight training needs and assist with quality assurance programmes.

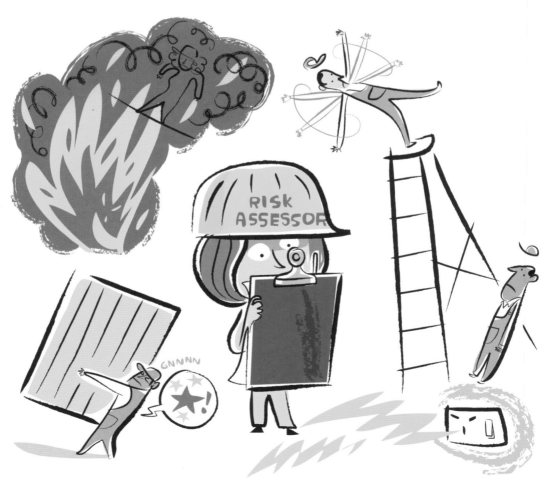

Hazards and risks

To discover how risk assessment works, it is important to understand the terms 'hazard' and 'risk'.

Hazards

A hazard is anything with the potential to cause harm. A range of hazards can be found in any workplace. Examples include:

- fire
- electricity
- harmful substances
- sharp instruments
- noise
- damaged flooring.

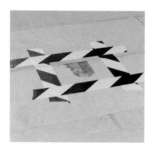

Damaged flooring is a hazard – it has the potential to cause harm

Risks

A risk is the likelihood that a hazard will cause harm. Risk depends on a number of factors. For example, the risk of tripping on a damaged floor surface will depend on:

- the extent of damage
- the number of people walking over it
- the number of times they walk over it
- whether they are wearing sensible shoes
- the level of lighting.

Control measures

Hazards in the workplace should be removed whenever possible. Using the example of the damaged floor, this would mean repairing the damage. Sometimes, however, there is no alternative but to keep a hazard. In such cases, it is important to reduce the risk – the likelihood of an accident – by introducing appropriate control measures. In the example about the floor, this could include placing a barrier around the damage or putting up warning signs.

Carrying out risk assessments

Everyone carries out informal risk assessments every day. For example, before crossing a road, we stop and look. We estimate the speed of the traffic and consider factors such as bad weather and poor visibility. On occasions, we may decide that it is too dangerous to cross at that place at that time and we may move to a pedestrian crossing where risks, such as traffic speed and visibility problems, may be reduced.

In health and social care settings staff may be expected to lift heavy loads with or without mechanical aids. It is important that detailed risk assessments are carried out to establish the safest approach to the task.

Formal risk assessments must be carried out in every workplace. The assessors are usually specially trained, competent managers and supervisors who are familiar with the task or issue being assessed and suitable safety controls. They must also be up-to-date with relevant legal requirements. Risk assessments must only be conducted by a competent person. Some tasks may require specialised risk assessments – for example, portable appliance testing – conducted by specialist risk assessors.

The risk assessment process involves analysing tasks carefully to estimate the nature and level of hazards and risks. Staff are often asked to become involved in the process.

There are a number of stages to carrying out a risk assessment and the people involved need to find answers to the following questions:

What are the hazards?

The workplace and activities must be carefully examined. Some hazards will be obvious, such as cables trailing across a gangway. Others may be hidden, such as those associated with manual handling.

Who is at risk?

Everyone or only certain people in an area may be at risk. For example, the risk of infection may affect everyone in a unit or ward or only those in close contact with an infected patient. Some groups of people may need special safety consideration as they may be more vulnerable to certain hazards – for example, pregnant women may be particularly at risk when lifting heavy objects, while young people may not be aware of all the workplace hazards and the need to follow safe procedures.

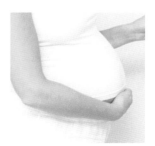

Specific risk assessments should be carried out for pregnant women and young persons

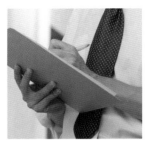

Formal risk assessments must be carried out in every workplace

How big is the risk?

Three questions are necessary here:

1. What are the consequences of injury or harm?

The consequences could range from a scratch to a death. The most severe hazards need the most urgent attention.

2. What is the likelihood of injury or harm?

Something that is very likely will need remedying before something that is unlikely.

3. How many people are affected?

Fire in a building could possibly harm everyone, but a trailing cable in an office might only affect one or two people.

Can we introduce additional control measures?

Where a hazard or risk is not already adequately controlled, it may be possible to introduce extra measures. Various types may be used, although it is always best to remove a hazard if this is possible. For example, it would be better to repair a damaged floor surface, so removing a tripping hazard, than to leave the surface as it is and put up a warning sign.

It is not always possible to remove a hazard, but it may be possible to separate people from it – for example, a bed rail bumper, placed over bed rails, can help a patient/client from trapping his/her legs. Sometimes it is possible to make a substitution, such as by replacing a dangerous cleaning chemical with a less hazardous one.

As a last resort, staff may be provided with personal protective equipment (PPE). For example, barrier clothing and gloves to protect a person from hazardous substances (chemical or biological). However, it is important to remember that the hazard is not sufficiently controlled, even though people are protected.

All control measures must be checked on a regular basis to ensure that they are working effectively.

What other action is needed?

Information and training on all hazards and control measures must be provided. Records of the assessments should be kept.

Risk assessments must be reviewed from time to time to ensure that the control measures continue to be appropriate. A review should always take place when changes are made, such as the introduction of new equipment. Managers and staff who carry out risk assessments need full training in the technique and the legal requirements.

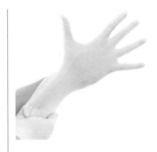

As a last resort, staff may be provided with PPE

Key points

- Risk assessment is an important technique that helps to prevent accidents and ill health.

- Risk assessment encourages managers and key staff to think about what could go wrong so that they can control the situation before accidents or ill health occurs.

- A thorough risk assessment programme can help to improve operational efficiency, offer financial savings and maintain professional reputations.

Summary

1. A hazard is anything with the potential to cause harm.

2. A risk is the likelihood that that a hazard will cause harm.

3. Control measures can help to reduce risk.

4. Risk assessment is an important technique that helps to prevent accidents and ill health.

5. Risk assessment encourages managers and key staff to think about what could go wrong so that they can control the situation before accidents or ill health occurs.

6. A thorough risk assessment programme can help to improve operational efficiency, offer financial savings and maintain professional reputations.

Chapter 4
Health

Some dangers, such as trapping a hand in moving machinery, are easy to spot, but many health problems develop gradually. For example, staff may breathe in dangerous substances or be exposed to radioactivity that eventually cause respiratory and other problems or they may strain their arms or back from working in a badly-arranged environment. As many occupational health problems are irreversible, it is important to consider the possibility of health hazards in order to prevent them from causing illness and disease.

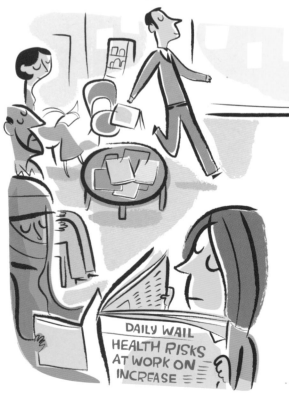

Key words

Acute – an effect on the body that occurs rapidly after a short exposure to a health hazard.

Carcinogen – a substance that can cause cancer in humans.

Chronic – an effect on the body that occurs after a long period of exposure or after repeated exposure.

Exposure – contact with a health hazard.

Health hazard – anything with the potential to cause ill health.

Hierarchy of controls – control measures listed in order of priority.

Occupational health – the activity of predicting and preventing work-related ill health. Also, health issues associated with work.

Health hazards

There are various types of health hazard:

- **chemical** – such as harmful dusts and liquids
- **biological** – such as infectious diseases
- **physical** – such as noise, heat and radiation
- **ergonomic** – such as badly-designed tasks, areas and equipment.

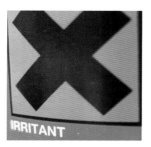

Chemical health hazards include cleaning fluids

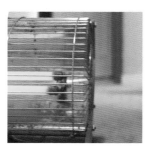

Heaters can pose physical health hazards

Effects on health

The effects of occupational health hazards may be acute – occurring shortly after exposure to a hazard – or they may be chronic – occurring after a long period of exposure or after repeated exposure. Harmful effects include:

- skin diseases, such as dermatitis
- respiratory diseases, such as silicosis
- suffocation, such as through carbon monoxide poisoning
- cancer due to contact with a carcinogen such as asbestos
- disorders of the central nervous system
- damage to body organs
- blood-borne infections
- birth defects as a result of contact with certain substances that damage human genes
- heat stroke through working in high-temperature environments
- work-related upper limb disorder, such as through repetitive movements
- work-related stress.

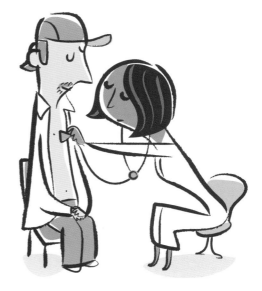

There are a number of ways in which hazardous substances can enter the body:

- **absorption** – where a hazardous substance gets onto the skin and is absorbed through it into the body and bloodstream.

- **ingestion** – through swallowing a hazardous substance or where one might be splashed into the mouth.

- **inhalation** – through breathing in a hazardous substance, such as toxic fumes.

- **injection** – where a sharp object, such as a needle, has a hazardous substance on it and cuts or punctures the skin.

The human body has many defences to prevent the entry of harmful substances. These include the skin and linings of the airways and gut. There are also defence mechanisms, such as coughing, sneezing, diarrhoea and vomiting, to expel harmful substances, while mucus and tears can trap particles or wash them away. Nonetheless, highly toxic substances, or high, long or repeated exposure, may cause illness and disease.

Key points

- Health hazards may cause a variety of effects, including diseases of the skin and lungs, bodily damage and disorders.

- Substances can enter the body by absorption, ingestion, inhalation and injection.

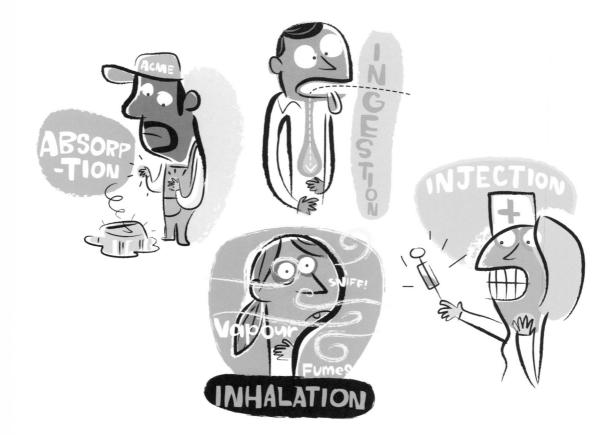

Preventing ill health from workplace hazards

It is important to identify occupational health hazards and to prevent them whenever possible. Good practice involves:

- identifying and avoiding health hazards

- measuring and assessing the hazards and risks

- applying control measures, such as good design, safe working procedures and/or the use of personal protective equipment/clothing

- regular reviews to check for changes.

Health hazards must be identified whether they are within the workplace or associated with work activities. If possible, hazards should be avoided altogether. Where this is not reasonably practicable, managers or proprietors must measure the extent of the hazard and risks. This may involve complex techniques and comparisons. In certain cases, there are government-set levels that must not be exceeded.

Appropriately qualified and experienced professionals may need to be consulted for advice, such as an ergonomist or occupational hygienist.

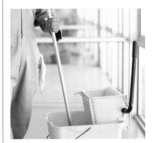

If health hazards cannot be avoided, control measures must be applied

Key point

- To prevent ill health caused by workplace hazards it is important to:

  - identify and avoid health hazards
  - measure and assess hazards and risks
  - apply control measures
  - review regularly to check for changes.

Control measures

If the hazard cannot be avoided, control measures must be put in place to minimise the likelihood of harmful effects and their consequences.

Some types of control measure are more effective than others. For example, a first and more effective measure might be to replace (substitute) a highly toxic cleaning chemical for a less hazardous one, but it may still be necessary to use gloves, goggles and other personal protective equipment. Nonetheless, this is better than continuing to use the original chemical while relying on personal protective equipment.

The list below shows various types of control measure. They are listed in order of priority and are sometimes referred to as the 'hierarchy of controls':

1. **Elimination** – can the hazard be eliminated?

If not, then:

2. **Substitution** – providing a safer alternative.

3. **Isolation** – moving a process to another area.

4. **Enclosure** – physically separating a process.

5. **Local ventilation** – removing the hazard directly from the process.

6. **General ventilation** – using normal room ventilation to reduce the hazard.

7. **Good housekeeping** – reducing risks from spills, dust and debris.

8. **Exposure time reduction** – reducing the time that people spend in contact with the hazard.

9. **Training** – to help individuals to reduce risks.

10. **Personal protective equipment** – to protect people on an individual basis.

11. **Welfare facilities** – to assist in minimising the risk, such as washing facilities.

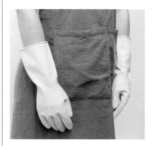

Personal protective equipment/clothing can protect people on an individual basis

Health surveillance and medical testing may also be necessary to detect early signs of ill health and to identify anyone who is particularly susceptible to a hazard and may need special consideration. Surveillance and testing can help to indicate the effectiveness of the control measures but should not be relied upon as proper safety controls because they can only detect – not prevent – ill health.

First aid and emergency facilities must also be provided. Again, these should not be relied upon as safety controls, although early treatment of symptoms will help to reduce harmful effects.

Staff should be given training in work-based hazards and risks and in the measures necessary to protect themselves and others. They also need to know about the possible harmful effects of their activities and to understand that they must report the first symptoms immediately.

Other management practices, such as regular inspections, supervision, good communication, maintenance and the identification of changes in the workplace or work tasks, must also be carried out to ensure that the control measures continue to reduce hazards and risks to an acceptable level.

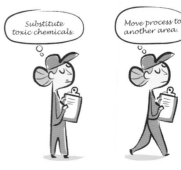

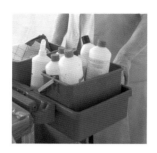

Good housekeeping can help to reduce risks from spills, dust and debris

Key points

- Control measures must be applied where health hazards cannot be avoided.

- If the hazard cannot be eliminated, then other measures must be considered, such as:

  – substitution

  – isolation and enclosure

  – ventilation

  – good housekeeping

  – exposure time reduction

  – training

  – personal protective equipment

  – welfare facilities.

- Health surveillance can be used to detect ill health and indicate the effectiveness, or otherwise, of control measures.

Summary

1. Health hazards can be chemical, biological, physical or ergonomic.

2. Health hazards may cause a variety of effects, including diseases of the skin and lungs, bodily damage and disorders.

3. Substances can enter the body by absorption, ingestion, inhalation or injection

4. To prevent ill health caused by workplace hazards it is important to:

   - identify and avoid health hazards
   - measure and assess hazards and risks
   - apply control measures
   - review regularly to check for changes.

5. Control measures must be applied where health hazards cannot be avoided.

6. If the hazard cannot be eliminated, then other measures must be considered, such as:

   - substitution
   - isolation and enclosure
   - ventilation
   - good housekeeping
   - exposure time reduction
   - training
   - personal protective equipment
   - welfare facilities.

7. Health surveillance can be used to detect ill health and indicate the effectiveness, or otherwise, of control measures.

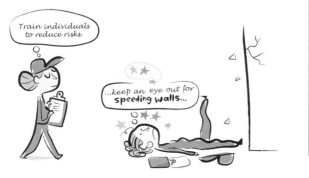

Chapter 5
Safety – accident prevention

An accident is an unplanned, uncontrolled event, which may cause major or minor injury, disease, illness, death, damage or other loss, such as delays incurring overtime costs or increased waiting times for some treatments. Safety is about not having accidents and reducing the risk of accidents and injury by putting in place appropriate control measures.

There are a number of ways in which people can be harmed through poor safety: electricity, fire and slips, trips and falls are three different aspects of safety that can all harm people in certain ways (*see* Chapters 6–8). In Great Britain, a system has been developed whereby certain accidents are reported centrally so that it is known where the greatest risks are and what the best way is of reducing them.

Key words

Accident – an unplanned, uncontrolled event with the potential to cause injury, damage or other loss.

Control or control measure – an item or action designed to remove a hazard or reduce the risk from it.

Reportable accident – an accident that must be reported to the appropriate enforcement authority.

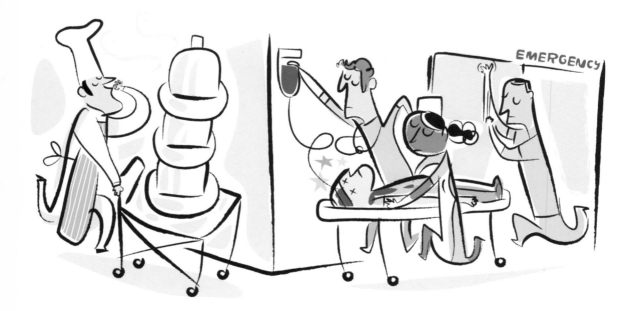

Accident prevention

There are always reasons why accidents occur – they do not just 'happen'. It is, therefore, essential to:

- examine the workplace and all its activities to assess what could go wrong
- select safety controls to prevent accidents from happening
- examine what has caused accidents in the past and why
- implement health and safety measures and check them regularly to ensure that they remain effective.

Risk assessment can help prevent accidents by:

- identifying what can harm people and how
- assessing the existing control measures
- seeing if there is anything more that can be done to reduce the risk of harm.

Accidents where people escape injury are commonly called 'near-misses'. These should also be investigated to help to develop measures that will prevent future injuries. This is of particular importance within the health and social care sector where sharing such knowledge may result in the prevention of accidents across a broad spectrum of activities and premises.

Accident statistics

Accident statistics can be viewed as a triangle. The accident triangle shows the relative number of outcomes of accidents at work – from the rare accidents resulting in death to the most common incidents, or near misses, resulting in no injury. It is important to recognise that some of the situations that lead to incidents *without* injury could also lead to an accident *with* injury.

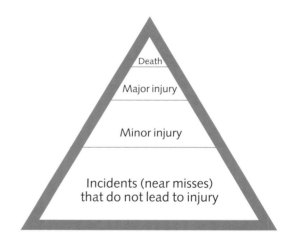

- Death
- Major injury
- Minor injury
- Incidents (near misses) that do not lead to injury

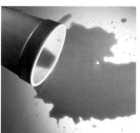

Near misses should also be investigated

Causes of accidents

The following examples show how accidents can be caused:

1. A cleaner badly cuts his finger when removing a bin liner that contains a scalpel

Possible causes – the cleaner:

- was using an unsafe working practice
- had not been properly trained.

Another member of staff:

- used the wrong bin to dispose of the scalpel.

2. An elderly client falls down the steps of a day centre, causing neck and spinal injuries

Possible causes:

- the centre was badly designed
- the manager had not allocated care staff to supervise the client properly
- the client was confused
- there was no handrail and the steps were steep.

3. A hospital worker injures her back when lifting a patient

Possible causes:

- the employer had failed to carry out an effective risk assessment for this process
- insufficient space around the patient's bed (poor workplace design)
- adequate hoists or lifting equipment were not supplied
- proper training had not been given in safe lifting techniques
- the member of staff had failed to follow safe working practices
- poor communication between staff prior to the procedure
- pressure of work and inadequate staffing levels.

Manual handling accidents can result in injury to staff and patients or clients. For example, a stand hoist requires that the patient has two functioning hands and arms and can support themselves as the hoist stands them. It has a strap that goes around the torso of the patient and, if the strap is not on properly or too high or the patient cannot hold on to hoist, they may be in danger of asphyxiation.

Two members of staff are needed to use a stand hoist and it is only suitable for patients with some mobility (not those with paralysis or generalised weakness). It is possible for a patient to experience a respiratory arrest on a stand hoist if used incorrectly.

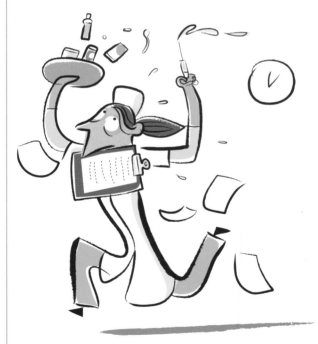

Factors contributing to accidents

Many situations and actions can cause accidents, and a combination of several factors often leads to accidents that end in serious injury.

Factors that contribute to accidents at work include:

- poor design and structure of buildings
- poorly designed, selected, constructed, guarded or maintained equipment
- bad housekeeping standards, such as blocked corridors and spilled liquids
- poor lighting or ventilation
- lack of information, instruction, training and supervision
- dangerous working practices
- distractions and lack of attention
- playing games or practical jokes
- the use of alcohol or drugs, or both
- working while ill or tired
- no or poor supervision
- working too quickly
- ignoring rules
- wearing unsuitable clothing
- not wearing the correct personal protective equipment/clothing (PPE/C).

Key point

- Many factors contribute to accidents, and a combination of several factors often leads to accidents that end in serious injury.

Accident reporting

Employers need to know that accidents have occurred so that they can prevent them from happening again. All accidents, including near-misses, and all health problems must be reported to supervisors or managers immediately by following the reporting procedure in the organisation. The management should then investigate the accident or circumstances to discover the cause, and set up appropriate controls to prevent health or safety problems from recurring.

All the important points about the accident, near-miss or instance of ill health must be noted in an accident book. The information is needed for the investigation and also provides a written record.

Some accidents must be reported to the enforcement authorities. They include accidents that result in:

- a death
- any type of injury, dangerous occurrence or disease that is specified by law
- an injury resulting in absence from work for more than three days
- a member of the public needing to go to hospital immediately.

Employers, the self-employed and others with the responsibility for reporting incidents should familiarise themselves with the relevant reporting requirements.

Key points

- All accidents and work-related health problems, including near-misses and violence or the threat of it, must be reported to employers or the person in charge.
- Investigating accidents, near-misses and work-related health problems helps in the development of measures to prevent recurrences.
- Records must be kept of all accidents, near-misses and work-related health problems.
- Certain accidents must be reported to the enforcement authorities.

Co-operation and communication

The management of health and safety standards and the behaviour of everyone in an organisation both play crucial parts in preventing accidents and ill health. It is important that managers make health and safety one of their priorities and take the lead on establishing good practices. However, high standards cannot be achieved unless everyone in an organisation takes health and safety seriously. Everyone at work must, therefore, follow health and safety instructions and training and report any defects or problems. In this way, employees are then reliant on each other for their safety and well-being.

Some staff, such as safety representatives, are given additional safety responsibilities. Good communication between staff and management is essential and there are legal requirements for consultation and safety committees. Managers should consult staff during risk assessments and when plans are made for changes, such as re-designing the workplace.

Organisations with good health and safety records often use a variety of techniques to involve staff in health and safety issues. These include formal communications through a safety committee and informal day-to-day discussions.

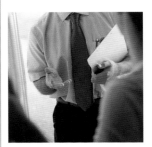

Good communication between management and staff is essential

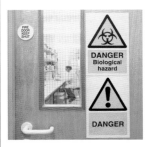

Everyone at work must follow health and safety instructions

Key point

■ Measures to help to prevent accidents and ill health include:

– examining the workplace and work activities to anticipate the causes of accidents

– controlling the environment, activities and specific hazards

– encouraging co-operation between everyone in a workplace

– following instructions and using safe procedures.

Summary

1. There are always reasons why accidents occur – they do not just 'happen'.

2. Many factors contribute to accidents, and a combination of several factors often leads to accidents that end in serious injury.

3. All accidents and work-related health problems, including near-misses and violence or the threat of it, must be reported to employers or the person in charge.

4. Investigating accidents, near-misses and work-related health problems helps in the development of measures to prevent recurrences.

5. Records must be kept of all accidents, near-misses and work-related health problems.

6. Certain accidents must be reported to the enforcement authorities.

7. Measures to help to prevent accidents and ill health include:

- examining the workplace and work activities to anticipate the causes of accidents

- controlling the environment, activities and specific hazards

- encouraging co-operation between everyone in a workplace

- following instructions and using safe procedures.

Chapter 6
Safety – slips, trips and falls

Everyone is exposed to the risk of slipping, tripping and falling regardless of where they work. Slips, trips and falls account for over a third of all reported accidents at work and are the primary cause of major classified accidents to workers. Slips, trips and falls are also a risk to the public, causing 50% of all accidents. In health and social care facilities, the risks of slips, trips and falls are heightened because of the vulnerability of patients/clients, the use of portable equipment and the greater likelihood of fluid spillages.

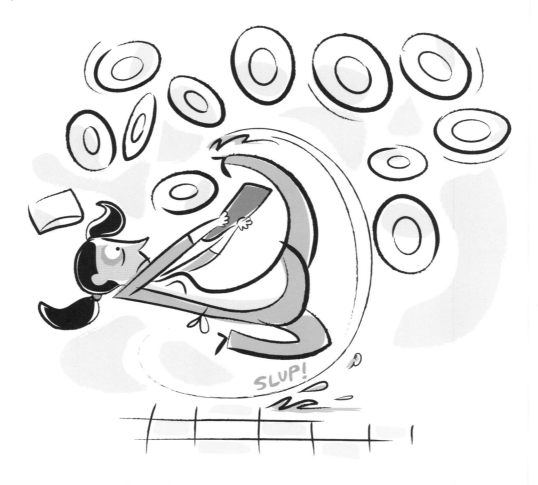

Key words

Fall – where a slip or a trip causes a person who was upright (walking or running) to fall to the ground or floor surface.

Slip – a term used to describe where the surface of footwear (or the sole of the foot) loses grip with the floor surface.

Trip – where an obstruction or uneven surface causes the foot or leg to 'catch' the obstruction, making a person lose balance.

Causes of slips, trips and falls

The main reasons for slips, trips and falls include:

- wet floors – failure to identify hazardous areas
- poor cleaning routines
- highly polished floors
- stairs that are damaged; in particular, the tread (flat surface) and the nosing (the very front edging of a step)
- obstructions and things left lying around on the floor
- trailing cables and wires, particularly portable medical equipment
- cleaning materials and equipment left out
- worn carpets, rugs and mats placed in the wrong place
- floor surfaces that are holed, cracked, uneven or damaged in some other way
- poor lighting
- wearing the wrong type of footwear
- people's behaviour, e.g. running instead of walking, carrying too much and obstructing the view ahead (which is more of a risk on stairs)
- using chairs instead of stepladders or proper foot stools.

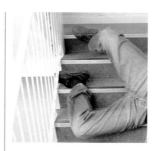

Walk don't run

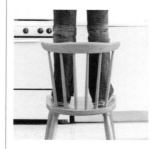

Use a step ladder or proper foot stool not a chair

Elderly patients and clients are at particular risk from falls. Over one third of over 65s are likely to experience a falling accident. Elderly women are at a higher risk than men. The stance and gait of men makes them generally more stable.

Other factors contributing to the risk of falls include:

- medication
- badly-fitting clothing and footwear
- confusion or debilitation.

For example, an elderly and confused patient may be able to manouver to the side of the bed but when he tries to stand, he is are unable to support his own weight and falls.Patients with confusion or memory loss require a great deal of supervision and regular reminders to use the call bell to summon help when they want to move.

In some cases, it may be appropriate to use beds with constraining rails, but this option needs to be individually assessed. The use of constraining rails may cause further distress to confused patients and could result in greater injury if they attempt to climb over the rails and fall from an even greater height.

The key to preventing falls is efficient risk assessment. Risk assessments must be regularly reviewed and, if necessary, updated and, of course, care staff need to read them.

Key point

- Slips, trips and falls are a major risk and cause of accidents.

Control measures

Slips are very difficult to control in certain environments where – for hygiene reasons – floors are smooth and may become slippery.
The HSE has produced a slips assessment tool (SAT) to help to identify risk areas. Equipment is also available that can measure how slippery a surface is by measuring its 'roughness'.

Most measures to prevent slips trips and falls are fairly simple and include:

- maintaining floors and floor surfaces in good condition
- keeping floors free from obstruction through good housekeeping
- covering or re-routing cables and wiring
- maintaining the premises and equipment to prevent leaks of water and fluids
- mopping up spillages as soon as they are spotted
- putting up warning notices and signs
- good lighting and having adequate space to do jobs
- wearing the correct footwear, including anti-slip soles for some workplaces
- putting in place rules to follow for workers and the public, such as no running and reporting of any slip or trip hazards they might spot.

While ensuring that floor surfaces and all environmental factors are as good as possible to prevent slips, trips and falls, much is down to human behaviour. If there are certain rules in place, such as no running or to wear a certain type of slip-resistant footwear, the advice MUST be followed. Otherwise, you may be prosecuted or disciplined by your employer; worse still, you may have an accident.

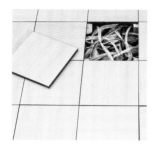

Cables and wires should be routed to prevent tripping

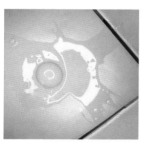

Mop up spillages as soon as they are spotted

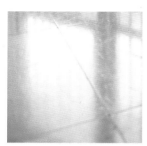

Maintaining floors and floor surfaces in good condition

Key points

- Good housekeeping is one of the best ways to reduce the risk of slips, trips and falls.

- Floors and stairs need to be kept in good condition and be well lit.

- Good, appropriate footwear needs to be worn and in certain areas, this will include footwear with anti-slip soles.

Summary

1. Slips, trips and falls are a major risk and cause of accidents.

2. Good housekeeping is one of the best ways to reduce the risk of slips, trips and falls.

3. Floors and stairs need to be kept in good condition and be well lit.

4. Good, appropriate footwear needs to be worn and in certain areas, this will include footwear with anti-slip soles.

Chapter 7
Safety – electricity

Electricity can cause electric shock, burns, fires and death. The fatality rate from injuries caused by electricity is high. It is, therefore, essential that electrical systems and equipment are designed, constructed, selected, maintained and used with care. Electricity is used in virtually every workplace – and even our safety systems may involve the use of electricity – so everyone must use electricity in the safest possible way.

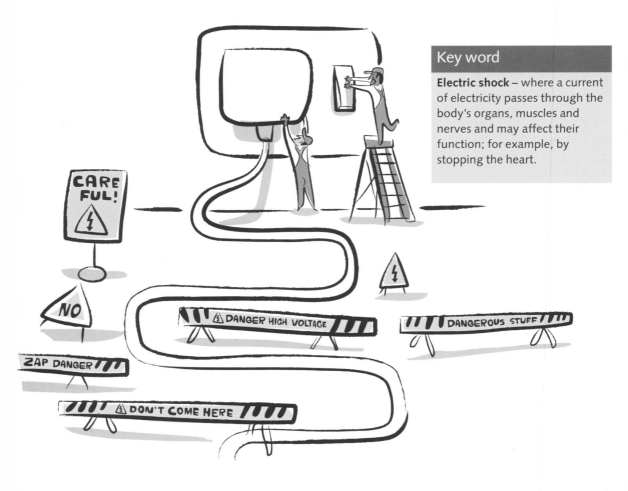

Key word

Electric shock – where a current of electricity passes through the body's organs, muscles and nerves and may affect their function; for example, by stopping the heart.

Reducing the risks from electricity

It may be possible to remove an electrical hazard by using a manual tool. If it is not feasible to avoid the hazard or substitute equipment, it is important to find appropriate controls to improve electrical safety. Such controls could involve:

- **insulation** – to protect people against direct contact with electricity

- **earthing** – to provide a connection to earth, so protecting against contact with electricity

- **fuses** – protective strips of metal that melt and break if overheating occurs, stopping the supply of electricity and preventing overheating and fire

- **circuit breakers** – to detect excess flow of electrical current and stop the electricity supply to the circuit, provided that they are of the correct type and rating

- **residual current circuit breakers** – to protect against electric shock

- **voltage reduction** – so that the lowest possible voltage is used.

In addition, all cables, plugs and sockets must be suitable for their use.

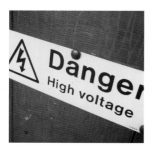

The fatality rate from injuries caused by electricity is high

Design, construction and selection

If you are involved in selecting and purchasing electrical equipment, you should consider the following points:

- whether the design and construction suits the purpose required, especially the likely degree of wear and tear

- whether the item is designed to suit the environment in which it will be used, e.g. specially designed and constructed equipment is needed in wet or explosive conditions

- whether it complies with legal requirements

- possible additional risks from second-hand equipment

- the need to avoid adapters and trailing cables when the item is installed or in use.

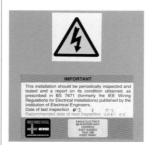

Electrical equipment must comply with legal requirements

Key point

- Equipment must be well designed and constructed and appropriate for its use. It must be installed safely and maintained and tested regularly.

Use of competent personnel

It is essential that systems are installed, checked regularly and maintained by competent, suitably qualified electricians or electrical engineers. You should never tamper with electrical equipment, attempt to repair it or remedy an electrical problem unless you have had specific training and have been authorised to do so. Qualified electricians must follow special procedures to prevent danger to themselves or to others.

Testing and maintenance

Equipment and systems that use electricity must be tested regularly and maintained thoroughly by competent personnel. The frequency of testing depends on a number of factors, such as the degree of wear and tear. Portable equipment requires extra attention.

Using electrical equipment

Organisations should establish safe working procedures, which should always be followed. Employers should ensure that employees receive full information, training and instruction on using electrical equipment safely and that they are supervised appropriately.

Always ensure that the power supply is turned off:
- when equipment is not in use (unless you have been instructed to leave it switched on)
- before opening, dismantling, maintaining or cleaning it
- when a fault, such as overheating, is evident or suspected
- before inserting a plug into a socket or removing it.

As water conducts electricity, you must ensure that you never:
- use electrical equipment in wet conditions (unless the equipment is specifically designed for the purpose)
- touch electrical equipment, switches, plugs or other electrical items with wet hands.

Although electrical equipment used in health and social care is manufactured to be used safely in adverse conditions, staff should always take precautions to ensure safety.

Key point

- General precautions include:
  - keeping the power supply disconnected when it is not required
  - keeping water and electricity apart
  - checking equipment before use and reporting defects immediately
  - using appropriate equipment for the task
  - using equipment according to the safety procedures of the workplace
  - using electrical equipment only if you have been trained and are authorised to use it.

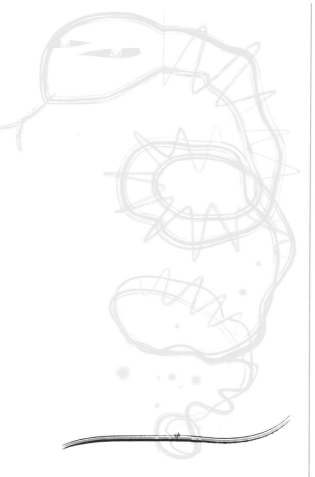

Reporting defects

Everyone who uses electrical equipment or works in an area where electricity is used must look out for problems and report them immediately. Some signs of a problem include:

- damaged sockets, plugs or cables
- evidence of overheating, such as burning smells or blackened sockets
- frequently blown fuses or electrical shocks.

Qualified and experienced personnel must then examine the equipment and make any necessary repairs or improvements.

Dealing with an emergency

A person who has received an electric shock may not be breathing and the heart may have stopped pumping blood around the body. The skin may be burned around the point of contact or the face may look pale or bluish, indicating that there may not be a pulse.

In the event of an emergency:

1. Seek help. One person can ring for the emergency services while another assists the casualty.

2. Do not put yourself in a position where you could be electrocuted. Do not touch the casualty, but try to switch the current off. If you cannot break the current, stand on dry insulating material and move the person away from the electrical source using material that does not conduct electricity, such as wood, plastic or wads of paper. However, do not attempt this if high voltage supplies, such as underground or overhead power lines, are involved.

3. If you are a qualified and competent first aider, follow your training for dealing with electric shock. If you are not qualified, carry out any instructions given by the first aider and ensure that any other people in the vicinity do not put themselves in danger.

4. Obtain emergency medical assistance for the casualty.

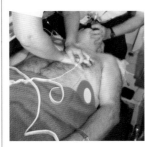

In the event of an emergency, seek help

Key point

■ In the event of an emergency, seek help and do not put yourself in a position where you could be electrocuted.

Legal requirements

There are legal requirements and official guidelines for the prevention of injury from electricity and the treatment of electric shock. Employers and the self-employed have a duty to assess what they need to do to comply with the requirements. Additional precautions may be needed for some activities and in some environments.

Employees have a legal duty to follow instructions and co-operate with their employer.

Key points

■ Employers and the self-employed have a duty to assess what they need to do to comply with legal requirements to prevent injury from electricity.

■ Employees have a duty to follow instructions and co-operate with their employer.

Summary

1. Electricity can cause electric shock, burns, fires and death.

2. The safety of electrical systems and equipment is improved by using insulation, earthing, fuses, circuit breakers, residual current circuit breakers and voltage reduction.

3. Equipment must be well designed and constructed and appropriate for its use. It must be installed safely and maintained and tested regularly.

4. General precautions include:

- keeping the power supply disconnected when it is not required

- keeping water and electricity apart

- checking equipment before use and reporting defects immediately

- using appropriate equipment for the task

- using equipment according to the safety procedures of the workplace

- using electrical equipment only if you have been trained and are authorised to use it.

5. In the event of an emergency, seek help and do not put yourself in a position where you could be electrocuted.

6. Employers and the self-employed have a duty to assess what they need to do to comply with legal requirements to prevent injury from electricity.

7. Employees have a duty to follow instructions and co-operate with their employer.

Chapter 8
Safety – fire prevention

Fire prevention is an important obligation for all organisations. Not only are people at work at risk from fire, but patients and clients, visitors, contractors, fire fighters, neighbours and anyone else in the vicinity may be affected.

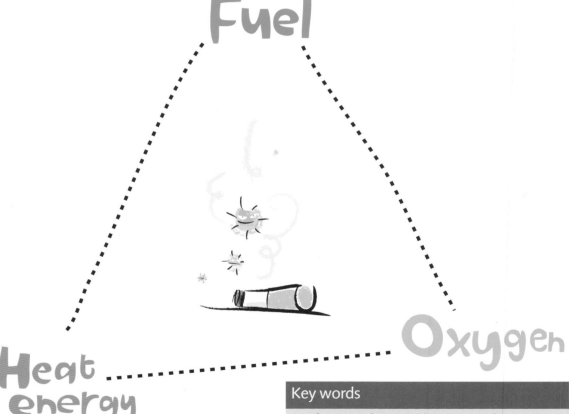

Fuel

Oxygen

Heat energy

Key words

Accelerant – substances that increase the rate at which a fire grows, such as oxygen.

Evacuation route – the designated way out of a building in case of fire or other emergency.

Fuel – anything that can be burned in a fire, such as paper, wood, furnishings and flammable chemicals.

Fire hazards and the causes of fires

The key hazards associated with fire are:

- flames and heat
- smoke and toxic fumes
- reduced oxygen
- collapse of buildings.

They may result in injury and death, possibly with many fatalities.

Fires may be caused in a variety of ways:

- sparks from electrical equipment
- overheated equipment
- hot surfaces, such as lighting and heating equipment
- tools or equipment with a naked flame
- hot liquids, such as fat in fryers
- smoking
- arson.

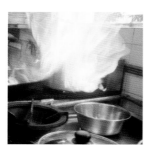

There are many potential causes of fire including hot liquids, such as fat

Key point

- Fire can cause damage, injury and death.

Fire prevention

Fire prevention and control depend on managing three factors, commonly referred to as the 'fire triangle' – fuel, oxygen and heat energy. Fires need the right combination of these three to burn.

Once a fire has started it may spread very quickly, producing smoke and toxic fumes. The emphasis must always be on preventing a fire from starting, rather than on putting it out. Fire risk assessments help employers to consider how to prevent fires.

Control of fuel

Material which could become fuel, either intentionally or by accident, must be kept to a minimum – for example, waste and rubbish should be removed regularly, the storage of flammable substances should be avoided or kept to the minimum and dusty atmospheres must be well ventilated. Fuel must be kept well away, and protected, from sources of ignition – for example, flammable substances must be kept in properly designed and selected fireproof stores or enclosures. Sources of ignition should be kept away from fuels – for example, smoking should be banned near stores of liquefied petroleum gas.

Control of oxygen

It is not usually possible to control the oxygen in the air, but fires can be put out by smothering them as this restricts the supply of oxygen that a fire needs to continue burning. The use of oxygen in health care environments carries a much enhanced risk of fire. All equipment must be regularly checked to prevent leakage and cylinders must be stored in a safe area, away from possible sources of ignition

Control of heat

Excessive heat and naked flames may start fires. These may be produced by friction in machines, hot surfaces, smoking, gas cookers and open fires.

Key point

- It is essential to maintain systems for fire prevention:

    - control sources of ignition

    - control fuels

    - avoid sources of ignition and fuels coming together.

Detectors and alarms

Detection systems are available which, when linked to a warning device, give early warning of a fire. The systems may detect high temperatures, smoke, radiation or certain gases produced by a fire. Manual or automatic fire alarms normally give the warning of danger by a loud sound, such as a ringing bell. Fire alarms must be checked regularly to make sure that they are working properly and everybody can hear them. Employees and regular users of a building should be made familiar with the sound of the fire alarm and the alarm signal should be explained to other people on their arrival.

Evacuation routes and procedures

All buildings must have a safe exit in case of fire. Emergency exits enable people to get out of a building in the opposite direction from a fire. Escape routes in large buildings need to be planned carefully so that they do not become too complicated.

Additional fire safety measures need to be installed in some buildings to protect the escape routes. These may include fire doors, emergency exits and fire resisting stair cases. Emergency exit doors must open outward to outdoors. They must not be locked unless strictly necessary. If they are locked, then there must be a safe emergency opening system that is labelled and explained.

Where elderly people or other vulnerable groups are present, particular care must be taken during the risk assessment process to ensure that they can be safely and swiftly removed from the building, in the event of a fire.

There must be permanent signposting that clearly shows the way out in an emergency. Escape routes and fire doors must be kept clear at all times. Internal fire doors must be kept closed as they help to prevent flames and smoke from spreading and limit the air supply to the fire.

There should also be an emergency lighting system that is checked regularly and maintained. Lifts must not be used as part of an evacuation route or during a fire because of the risk of people becoming trapped.

Managers need to know who is in a building, so staff, visitors and others should be asked to sign in and out. A register should be taken after evacuation to ensure that everyone has escaped.

Anyone who has to leave a building in an emergency should follow the instructions of the people in authority. Once evacuated, everyone should remain at the designated assembly point until told by someone in authority, such as a fire officer or senior manager, that it is safe to re-enter the building.

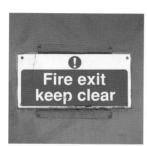

Escape routes must be kept clear at all times

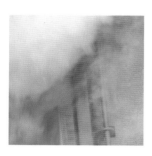

Internal fire doors help to prevent fire and smoke spreading

Key points

- Detection, warning and evacuation systems, routes and procedures must be carefully designed and maintained.

- All staff should be trained in fire procedures and other people should be briefed.

- Escape routes must be kept clear and be properly signposted.

- Fire doors should be kept closed.

- After evacuation, everyone should go to the designated assembly point where attendance should be checked. Nobody must re-enter a building until they have been told it is safe to do so.

Training and information

Everyone who uses a workplace should be trained what to do in case of a fire, explosion or other emergency. Where it is not possible to train people, such as visitors and contractors, a safety briefing should be given on their arrival.

Notices should be displayed at strategic points to give guidance on what to do in case of fire. Notices should describe the sound of the fire alarm, what to do when it sounds, what action to take on discovering a fire and where to assemble after leaving the building. Directions and diagrams should be provided in buildings where people may be unfamiliar with the layout.

Some staff may be nominated as fire wardens and given the responsibility for checking that everyone has been evacuated. They may be given extra training, such as fire fighting. On some premises, all staff must be trained in fire fighting because of the risk of fire or explosion.

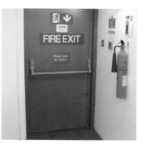

Notices should be displayed at strategic points to give guidance on what to do in case of fire

Key points

- Everyone who uses a workplace should be trained what to do in case of a fire, explosion or other emergency.

- Notices should be displayed at strategic points to give guidance on what to do in case of fire.

Fire drills

Regular fire drills should be carried out to check that the facilities and procedures are effective and that everyone understands what they should do. Remedial action must be taken if evacuation has been slow or incomplete.

As it is often impractical to carry out 'real-life' fire drills in health and social care settings, it is important that all staff be provided with training to ensure that they are fully aware of the procedures and systems in place to effect a safe evacuation of their work areas.

Fire fighting

It is more important to evacuate people from a building than to stop and fight a fire. However, there are occasions when simple fire-fighting techniques can eliminate a fire before it takes hold, such as when dealing with burning fat in a pan.

Fire-fighting techniques, which may be automatic or manual, eliminate one of the factors in the fire triangle, such as by:

- starving the fire of fuel
- restricting oxygen, e.g. by using a fire blanket to smother a pan of burning fat
- cooling the heat.

Sprinkler systems

These automatically detect and control a fire at an early stage. They need to be permanently connected to a water supply and must be properly designed and maintained.

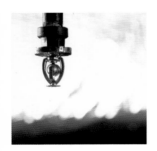

Sprinkler systems automatically detect and control fire at an early stage

Hose reels

These are normally provided for use by the fire brigade. They must be easily accessible and should not be tampered with

Portable fire extinguishers

It is important that any fire extinguisher used is of the correct type. Extinguishers are colour-coded and contain one of a number of substances that can put out fires:

- **water** – paper, wood, textile, solid material fires
- **powder** – liquid, electrical, wood, paper, textile fires
- **foam** – liquid, paper, wood, textile fires
- **carbon dioxide (CO_2)** – liquid and electrical fires

When operated, pressure releases the substance that can be directed onto the fire.

It is dangerous to attempt to tackle a fire unless you have been trained how to use an extinguisher and have made sure that you can get out of the building.

Portable fire extinguishers should be fixed in suitable, accessible positions – usually by doors along exit routes – and must be clearly indicated by specific safety signs. There should be enough of them for the type of premises and risks involved in the work activities. Extinguishers must be regularly checked and maintained by competent people.

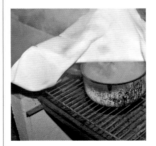

Simple fire fighting techniques can eliminate a fire before it takes hold

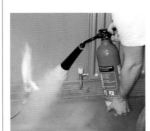

Do not use a fire extinguisher unless you have been trained

Fire extinguishers

Category	Type
Water	[A]
Powder	[A] [B] [C]
Foam	[A] [B]
CO₂	[B]

Key point

- It is dangerous to attempt to tackle a fire unless you have been trained how to use an extinguisher and have made sure that you can get out of the building.

Legal requirements

Various laws cover fire precautions and in Britain, some premises must hold a fire certificate. Employers, the self-employed and those in charge of buildings must familiarise themselves with the requirements that affect them. Advice can be obtained from enforcement authorities – in particular, the local fire authority.

Summary

1. Fire can cause damage, injury and death.

2. It is essential to maintain systems for fire prevention:

   - control sources of ignition

   - control fuels

   - avoid sources of ignition and fuels coming together.

3. Detection, warning and evacuation systems, routes and procedures must be carefully designed and maintained.

4. All staff should be trained in fire procedures and other people should be briefed.

5. Escape routes must be kept clear and be properly signposted.

6. Fire doors should be kept closed.

7. After evacuation, everyone should go to the designated assembly point where attendance should be checked. Nobody must re-enter a building until they have been told it is safe to do so.

8. Everyone who uses a workplace should be trained what to do in case of a fire, explosion or other emergency.

9. Notices should be displayed at strategic points to give guidance on what to do in case of fire.

10. It is dangerous to attempt to tackle a fire unless you have been trained how to use an extinguisher and have made sure that you can get out of the building.

Chapter 9
Welfare

Welfare is not just health and safety – it is about a person's well-being at work. Employers have to provide welfare facilities, such as toilets, washing facilities, drinking water and places to rest.

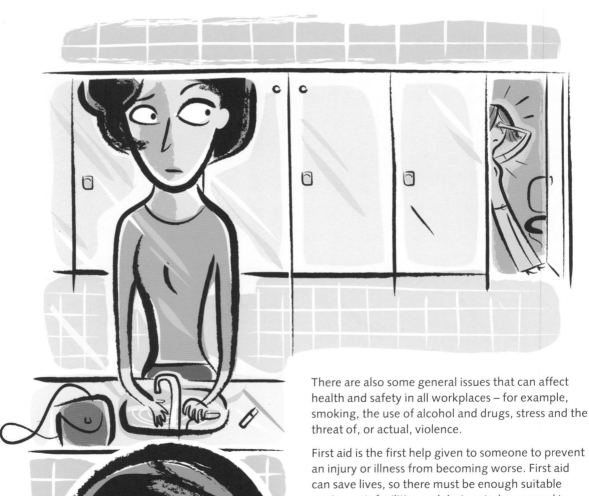

There are also some general issues that can affect health and safety in all workplaces – for example, smoking, the use of alcohol and drugs, stress and the threat of, or actual, violence.

First aid is the first help given to someone to prevent an injury or illness from becoming worse. First aid can save lives, so there must be enough suitable equipment, facilities and designated personnel in every workplace to deal with cases of injury or illness.

Key words

Appointed person – someone with specific duties relating to first aid, but not necessarily trained in first aid.

First aider – someone trained to a recognised standard to administer first aid.

Stress – a feeling of anxiety and unwanted pressure that causes harm to the body and a major cause of absenteeism at work.

Welfare – the provision of facilities and other measures to ensure a person's well-being.

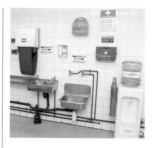

Employers must provide welfare facilities

Key point

- Welfare facilities are required to help maintain the well-being of persons at work.

Welfare facilities

Every workplace must provide:

- an adequate number of toilets that are kept clean, well lit and ventilated

- washing facilities with hot and cold water, soap and hand-drying facilities

- a supply of drinking water

- facilities for storing clothing and, where necessary, changing facilities

- facilities for staff during work breaks – this may mean providing seating, separate eating areas and smoking areas

- suitable rest facilities for pregnant women and nursing mothers.

Smoking

Smoke in the atmosphere can be considered a form of air pollution. Research has linked passive smoking to lung cancer in non-smokers, irritation of the respiratory system and other harmful effects. It is, therefore, important that everyone at work should comply with policies and restrictions on smoking – for example, by using only designated areas for smoking. In most health and social care settings, smoking is banned altogether. Where smoking is permitted, provision should be made for a separate area and consideration given to the use of non-combustible furniture, fittings, etc. The area should be properly ventilated and care taken to ensure that smoke does not affect others. The area should be supervised and regular checks made to ensure that the risk of fire is minimised.

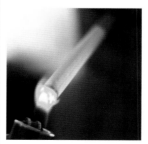

Smoking causes air pollution and has a harmful effect on smokers and non-smokers

Stress

Stress creates the production of hormones in the body which have physical effects. A certain amount of stress may help us to perform tasks to the best of our abilities, but excessive stress for long periods can cause tiredness, anxiety and various physical symptoms. Health problems that have been linked to stress include stomach and skin conditions, heart disease and depression.

Various factors have been shown to increase stress levels, such as working in poor or cramped conditions, lack of communication with managers, overworking, concern about the risk of injury or illness and lack of job security.

Employers can help to reduce stress levels by considering the causes and taking appropriate action, such as re-designing a job, improving working conditions, improving communication and providing support. Individuals may be able to help to decrease their stress levels by modifying their lifestyles and improving their fitness, while others may find relaxation techniques helpful.

Caring for sick and vulnerable people places great demands upon staff. If these pressures are not properly monitored and controlled, they can lead to stress. It is advisable to provide stress-awareness training for all personnel to help them identify the early signs of stress and to take the first steps to manage it effectively.

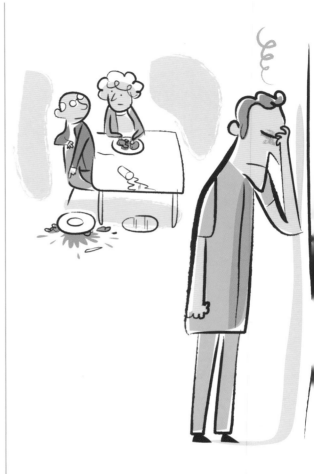

Alcohol

Alcohol increases the time taken to react to a situation, affects behaviour and reduces performance on jobs, such as driving or operating dangerous machinery.

Many employers have strict policies on alcohol and drugs – for example, staff may be banned from drinking at work, during breaks and before starting work. The policy may be supported by testing for alcohol with the employee's consent. It is important to remember that levels of alcohol in the body may still be high the morning after drinking the previous evening.

In health and social care environments, patients'/clients' lives may well depend upon the carers' abilities to think clearly and act promptly. It is for this reason that strict policies operate to sanction those who misuse alcohol.

Excessive alcohol consumption is normally viewed as a condition that can be treated, with the individual's co-operation, and employers may encourage people with a drink problem to seek professional help. However, as a last resort, employers may have to take disciplinary action, possibly even dismissing someone, to protect the drinker and others whose safety may be put at risk.

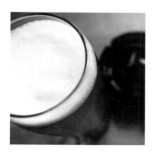

Alcohol can jeopardise the safety of an individual and his/her colleagues

Drugs

Substance abuse, the use of illegal drugs or the misuse of prescription drugs may cause health problems and can cause safety risks in the workplace. Many drugs are particularly dangerous because they can change people's moods and perceptions. It is important to check that prescribed drugs will not affect performance at work. If there is an increased risk to safety, staff should tell their manager or supervisor. Suitable arrangements can then be taken to protect everyone's safety.

Employers must not ignore drug abuse but should take action to help the person involved and to protect others from safety hazards that could occur as a result of the abuse.

Some workers, in the health and social care sectors, are at an increased risk of abuse and violence from patients or clients who are under the influence of drugs and/or alcohol. Workers' safety is paramount and should always be a priority.

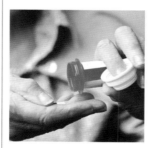

It is important to check that prescribed drugs will not affect your performance at work

Key point

- Alcohol and drugs have an adverse effect on the body, affecting judgement and increasing the risk of accidents and injury.

Violence

Verbal abuse, threats or assault can cause stress and anxiety as well as physical injury. Staff should always report violence, including verbal abuse, to their managers who should record and investigate the incident and, if necessary, report it to the relevant enforcement authority. As with other hazardous situations, employers and the self-employed should carry out risk assessments and put in place appropriate controls.

These could include measures such as improving the design of buildings to help create a more calming environment, giving staff training and information on how to deal with potentially difficult situations.

Lone workers

There are many areas of work within the health and social care sectors, where personnel are required to work alone. This may be with patients or clients on a one-to-one basis in an institution or when providing care in the community. Proper provision must be made to protect the safety and well-being of staff under these conditions. Training should be provided to help staff understand the hazards associated with lone working and to advise them of the systems in place to monitor and ensure their safety.

Key point

■ Employees who are subject to violence must report it.

Harassment and bullying

It is illegal under the Health and Safety at Work etc. Act, 1974, for an employee to bully or harass another employee. The effects of bullying cause those who are bullied a huge amount of anxiety or distress, which can often be one of the causes for absenteeism from work and contribute to stress.

A personal safety policy provides staff with a clear commitment, by management, to ensure that the organisation operates in such a way as to minimise the risks to staff in respect of verbal and non-verbal abuse. Bullying and harassment are both forms of abuse and must be eliminated from the workplace.

Key point

■ Harassment and bullying is illegal and can cause anxiety and stress.

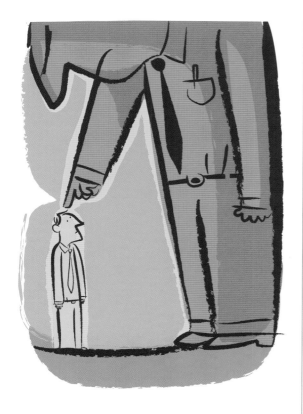

First aid provision

Risk assessments must be carried out to show the level of first aid provision needed. The minimum provision is a suitably stocked first aid kit and an 'appointed person' (*see* below). Various factors affect the level of risk and the requirements for first aid, such as:

- working with hazardous substances or dangerous equipment
- the number of people
- people with special needs or inexperienced workers
- work in remote areas
- work that involves regular travel
- lone or shift work
- interaction with staff from another company or organisation, or the presence of members of the public.

In some workplaces and circumstances, it may be necessary to provide more than the required minimum. For example, in care homes where elderly, young or other high-risk patients/clients may be present. This could involve training additional first aiders or providing extra first aid kits, mobile telephones or a first aid room. It may also be necessary to liaise with the emergency services – for example, to discuss special hazards.

Everyone at work must be made aware of first aid arrangements by instruction and notices.

First aid kits

The contents of a first aid kit should be linked to the risks at the site. Additional items may be needed where there are specific hazards – for example, eye-washing facilities may be needed where certain chemicals are handled. Medicines or tablets must never be kept in first aid kits because only qualified personnel are allowed to dispense them.

Minimum contents of a first aid box

The following items are recommended where there are no special risks:

- guidance leaflet
- 20 individually-wrapped, sterile, adhesive dressings of various sizes
- 2 sterile eye pads with attachments
- 6 individually-wrapped triangular bandages
- 6 safety pins
- 6 medium-sized, 2 large and 3 extra large individually-wrapped, sterile, unmedicated wound dressings
- 1 pair of disposable gloves (as required under HSE guidance).

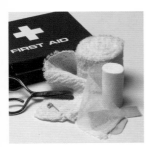

The contents of first aid kits vary according to workplace needs

Appointed persons and first aiders

An appointed person must be available whenever people are working. The responsibilities include looking after the first aid equipment, making sure it is always available, taking control when somebody is injured or ill and calling the emergency services if necessary. An appointed person does not have to be a trained first aider although basic training is recommended.

First aiders must be specially trained and certificated by organisations approved by the Health and Safety Executive. They should give treatment only in the techniques they have been trained to carry out; otherwise, they could cause further injury. First aiders may need additional training where there are special workplace hazards.

The numbers of appointed persons and first aiders needed in a workplace depend on factors such as risk, layout and number of employees, patients/clients and visitors.

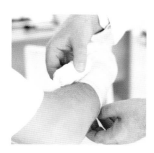

First aiders must be specially trained and certificated

Key points

- First aid prevents injury and illness from getting worse and can save lives.

- Adequate arrangements must be made for first aid, including responsible people, equipment and facilities.

- The exact first aid provision depends on the risks in the workplace.

- Employees should know what first aid arrangements have been made.

- Adequate numbers of trained first aiders should be available depending upon the risks in the workplace. The minimum provision of personnel is an appointed person.

Summary

1. Welfare facilities are required to maintain the well-being of persons at work.

2. Alcohol and drugs have an adverse effect on the body, affecting judgement and increasing the risk of accidents and injury.

3. Employees who are subject to violence must report it.

4. Harassment and bullying is illegal and can cause anxiety and stress.

5. First aid prevents injury and illness from getting worse and can save lives.

6. Adequate arrangements must be made for first aid, including responsible people, equipment and facilities.

7. The exact first aid provision depends on the risks in the workplace.

8. Employees should know what first aid arrangements have been made.

9. Adequate numbers of trained first aiders should be available depending upon the risks in the workplace. The minimum provision of personnel is an appointed person.

Index

Design: www.red-stone.com
Illustration: Ned Jolliffe

Photography: 3 (Zephyr/Science Photo Library), 7 (Altrendo Images/Altrendo/
Getty Images), 11 (Keith Brofsky/UpperCut Images), 13T (SHOUT/Alamy),
13M (SHOUT/Alamy), 17T (Paul Whitehill/Science Photo Library),
17B (MedioImages/Getty Images), 18 (Wide Group/Iconica/Getty Images),
21T (Image Source/Getty Images), 21B (Henry King/Photonica/Getty Images),
23 (George Doyle/Stockbyte Platinum/Getty Images), 24 (Image Source/
Getty Images), 25 (Altrendo Images/Altrendo/Getty Images), 27 (Nick Koudis/
Photodisc Green/Getty Images), 30T (Flying Colours Ltd/Digital Vision/
Getty Images), 30B (Steve Taylor/Digital Vision/Getty Images), 33T (Image
Source/Punchstock), 33B (Brandon Harman/Photonica/Getty Images),
35T (Martin Barraud/Stone/Getty Images), 35M (Firstlight/Getty Images),
35B (Image Source/Getty Images), 37L (Pixoi Ltd/Alamy), 37R (Andrew Olney),
40 (Stockbyte/Stockbyte Gold/Getty Images), 43 (Tim Hall/Photodisc Red/
Getty Images), 45LT (Pixoi Ltd/Alamy), 45LB (Michael Donne/Science Photo
Library), 45R (Andrew Olney), 46L (SuperStock/Alamy), 46RT (SHOUT/Alamy),
46RB (Cordelia Molloy/Science Photo Library), 49T (Andrew Olney),
49B (Bluestone/Science Photo Library), 51L (Ian Waldie/Reportage/Getty Images),
51R (Michael Goldman/Taxi/Getty Images), 54 (Dorling Kindersley/Getty Images),
55 (Stockbyte Platinum/Alamy)

Print: The Astron Group
Stock: Era Silk, 50% post-consumer waste and 50% TCF pulp